A Detailed Plant Based Diet Cookbook 2021

The Ultimate Plant Based Diet Cookbook,
Delicious Dishes Quick and Easy
to Prepare at Home for Losing Weight

John Becker

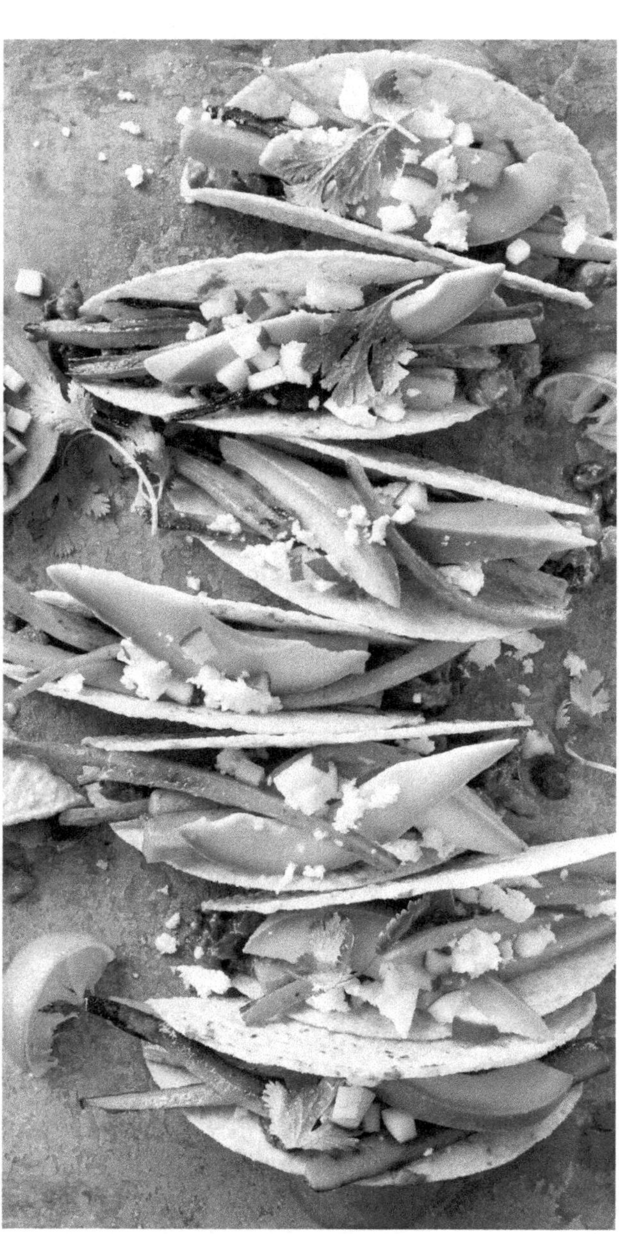

Table of Contents

The information in the following pages is broadly considered a truthful and accurate account of facts and as such, any inattention, use, or misuse of the information in question by the reader will render any resulting actions solely under their purview. There are no scenarios in which the publisher or the original author of this work can be in any fashion deemed liable for any hardship or damages that may befall them after undertaking information described herein.

Additionally, the information in the following pages is intended only for informational purposes and should thus be thought of as universal. As befitting its nature, it is presented without assurance regarding its prolonged validity or interim quality. Trademarks that are mentioned are done without written consent and can in no way be considered an endorsement from the trademark holder.

Introduction

A plant-based diet is a diet based primarily on whole plant foods. It is identical to the regular diet we're used to already, except that it leaves out foods that are not exclusively from plants. Hence, a plant-based diet does away with all types of animal-sourced foods, hydrogenated oils, refined sugars, and processed foods. A whole food plant-based diet comprises not just fruits and vegetables; it also consists of unprocessed or barely-processed oils with healthy monounsaturated fats (like extra-virgin olive oil), whole grains, legumes (essentially lentils and beans), seeds and nuts, as well as herbs and spices.

What makes a plant-based meal (or any meal) fun is the manner with which you make them; the seasoning process; and the combination process that contributes to a fantastic flavor and makes every meal unique and enjoyable. There are lots of delicious recipes (all plant-centered), which will prove helpful in when you intend making mouthwatering, healthy plant-based dishes for personal or household consumption. Provided you're eating these plant-based foods regularly, you'll have very problems with fat or diseases that result from bad dietary habits, and there would be no need for excessive calorie tracking.

Plant-based diet recipes are versatile; they range from colorful Salads to Lentil Stews, and Bean Burritos. The recipes also draw influences from around the globe, with Mexican, Chinese, European, Indian cuisines all part of the vast array of plant-based recipes available to choose from. Why You Ought to Reduce Your Intake of Processed and Animal-Based Foods. You have likely heard over and over that processed food has adverse effects on your health. You might have also been told repeatedly to stay away from foods with lots of preservatives; nevertheless, nobody ever offered any genuine or concrete facts about why you ought to avoid these foods and why they are unsafe. Consequently, let us properly dissect it to help you properly comprehend why you ought to stay away from these healthy eating offenders. They have massive habit-forming characteristics. Humans have a predisposition towards being addicted to some specific foods; however, the reality is that the fault is not wholly ours. Every one of the unhealthy treats we relish now and then triggers the dopamine release in our brains. This creates a pleasurable effect in our brain, but the excitement is usually short-lived. The discharged dopamine additionally causes an attachment connection gradually, and this is the reason some people consistently go back to eat certain unhealthy foods even when they know it's unhealthy and unnecessary.

You can get rid of this by taking out that inducement completely. They are sugar-laden and plenteous in glucose-fructose syrup. Animal-based and processed foods are laden with refined sugars and glucose-fructose syrup which has almost no beneficial food nutrient. An ever-increasing number of studies are affirming what several people presumed from the start; that genetically modified foods bring about inflammatory bowel disease, which consequently makes it increasingly difficult for the body to assimilate essential nutrients. The disadvantages that result from your body being unable to assimilate essential nutrients from consumed foods rightly cannot be overemphasized. Processed and animal-based food products contain plenteous amounts of refined carbohydrates. Indeed, your body requires carbohydrates to give it the needed energy to run body capacities. In any case, refining carbs dispenses with the fundamental supplements; in the way that refining entire grains disposes of the whole grain part. What remains, in the wake of refining, is what's considered as empty carbs or empty calories. These can negatively affect the metabolic system in your body by sharply increasing your blood sugar and insulin quantities. They contain lots of synthetic ingredients. At the point when your body is taking in non-natural ingredients, it regards them as foreign substances.

Your body treats them as a health threat. Your body isn't accustomed to identifying synthetic compounds like sucralose or these synthesized sugars. Hence, in defense of your health against this foreign "aggressor," your body does what it's capable of to safeguard your health. It sets off an immune reaction to tackle this "enemy" compound, which indirectly weakens your body's general disease alertness, making you susceptible to illnesses. The concentration and energy expended by your body in ensuring your immune system remain safe could instead be devoted somewhere else. They contain constituent elements that set off an excitable reward sensation in your body. A part of processed and animal-based foods contain compounds like glucose-fructose syrup, monosodium glutamate, and specific food dyes that can trigger some addiction. They rouse your body to receive a benefit in return whenever you consume them. Monosodium glutamate, for example, is added to many store-bought baked foods. This additive slowly conditions your palates to relish the taste. It gets mental just by how your brain interrelates with your taste sensors.

This reward-centric arrangement makes you crave it increasingly, which ends up exposing you to the danger of over consuming calories.

For animal protein, usually, the expression "subpar" is used to allude to plant proteins since they generally have lower levels of essential amino acids as against animal-sourced protein. Nevertheless, what the vast majority don't know is that large amounts of essential amino acids can prove detrimental to your health. Let me break it down further for you.

Pizza

Easy Flatbread Pizza

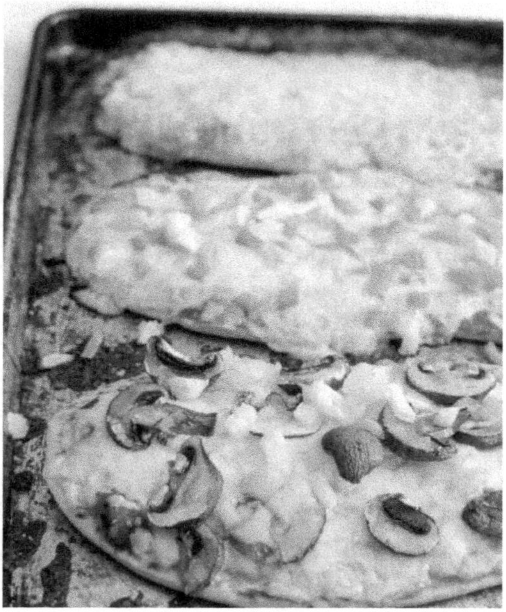

Preparation time: 10 minutes

Cooking time: 10 minutes

Servings: 3

Ingredients:

Nutrition: Calories 195, Carbs 23g, Fat 7g, Protein 9g

- Pita flatbread – 1

- Italian blend seasoning – 1/8 teaspoon.
- Red pepper flakes – 1/8 teaspoon.
- Cherry tomatoes – 1/2 cup, halved
- Mozzarella cheese – 1/2 cup, grated
- Pizza sauce – 3 tablespoons.

Directions:

1. Preheat the oven to 350 F. Spread pizza sauce, cheese, and cherry tomatoes over flatbread.
2. Sprinkle with red pepper flakes and Italian seasoning. Bake in a preheated oven for 10 minutes. Serve.

Creamy Squash Pizza

Preparation Time: 25 minutes

Cooking Time: 21 minutes

Serving: 4

Ingredients:

- 3 cups butternut squash, fresh or frozen, cubed
- 2 tbsp. minced garlic
- 1 tbsp. olive oil
- 1 tsp. red pepper flakes
- 1 tsp. cumin
- 1 tsp. paprika
- 1 tsp. oregano

Crust:

- 2 cups dry French green lentils
- 2 cups water
- 2 tbsp. minced garlic
- 1 tbsp. Italian seasoning
- 1 tsp. onion powder

Toppings:

- 1 tbsp. olive oil

- 1 medium green bell pepper, pitted, diced
- 1 cup chopped broccoli
- 1 small purple onion, diced

Directions:

1. Preheat the oven to 350°F.
2. Prepare the French green lentils according to the method.
3. Add all the sauce ingredients to a food processor or blender, and blend on low until everything has mixed and the sauce looks creamy. Set the sauce aside in a small bowl.
4. Clean the food processor or blender; then add all the ingredients for the crust and pulse on high speed until a dough-like batter has formed.
5. Heat a large deep-dish pan over medium-low heat and lightly grease it with 1 tablespoon of olive oil.
6. Press the crust dough into the skillet until it resembles a round pizza crust and cook until the crust is golden brown—about 5-6 minutes on each side.

7. Put the crust on a baking tray covered with parchment paper.
8. Coat the topside of the crust with the sauce using a spoon, and evenly distribute the toppings across the pizza.
9. Bake the pizza in the oven
10. Slice into 4 equal pieces and serve, or store.

Nutrition:

Calories 258, Total Fat 9.2g, Saturated Fat 1.2g, Cholesterol 2mg, Sodium 21mg, Total Carbohydrate 38.3g, Dietary Fiber 9.7g, Total Sugars 6.2g, Protein 9g, Vitamin D 0mcg, Calcium 111mg, Iron 4mg, Potassium 838mg

Fluffy Deep Dish Pizza

Preparation time: 10 minutes
Cooking time: 2 hours
Servings: 6
Ingredients:

- 12 inch of frozen whole-wheat pizza crust, thawed
- 1 medium-sized red bell pepper, cored and sliced
- 5-ounce of spinach leaves, chopped
- 1 small red onion, peeled and chopped
- 1 1/2 teaspoons of minced garlic
- 1/4 teaspoon of salt
- 1/2 teaspoon of red pepper flakes
- 1/2 teaspoon of dried thyme
- 1/4 cup of chopped basil, fresh
- 14-ounce of pizza sauce
- 1 cup of shredded vegan mozzarella

Directions:

1. Place a medium-sized non-stick skillet pan over an average heat, add the oil and let it heat.

2. Add the onion, garlic and let it cook for 5 minutes or until it gets soft.
3. Then add the red bell pepper and continue cooking for 4 minutes or until it becomes tender-crisp.
4. Add the spinach, salt, red pepper, thyme, basil and stir properly.
5. Cool off for 3 to 5 minutes or until the spinach leaves wilts, and then set it aside until it is called for.
6. Grease a 4-quarts slow cooker with a non-stick cooking spray and insert the pizza crust in it.
7. Press the dough into the bottom and spread 1 inch up along the sides.
8. Spread it with the pizza sauce, cover it with the spinach mixture and then garnish evenly with the cheese.
9. Sprinkle it with the red pepper flakes, basil leaves and cover it with the lid.
10. Plug in the slow cooker and let it cook for 1 1/2 hours to 2 hours at the low heat setting or until the crust turns golden brown and the cheese melts completely.

11. When done, transfer the pizza into the cutting board, let it rest for 10 minutes, then slice to serve.

Nutrition:

Calories: 250 Cal,

Carbohydrates: 25g,

Protein: 5g,

Fats: 8g,

Fiber: 1g.

Incredible Artichoke and Olives Pizza

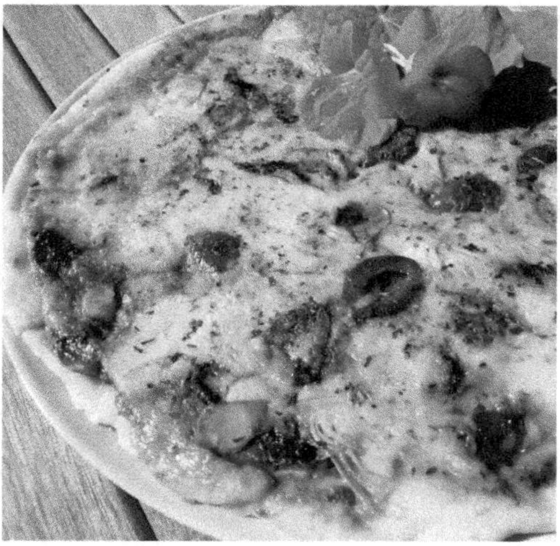

Preparation time: 20 minutes

Cooking time: 1 hour 50 minutes

Servings: 6

Ingredients:

- 12 inch of frozen whole-wheat pizza crust, thawed
- 1 mushroom, sliced
- 1/2 cup of sliced char-grilled artichokes
- 1 small green bell pepper, cored and sliced
- 2 medium-sized tomatoes, sliced
- 2 tablespoons of sliced black olives

- 1/2 teaspoon of garlic powder
- 1 teaspoon of salt, divided
- 1/2 teaspoon of dried oregano
- 2 tablespoons of nutritional yeast
- 2-ounce cashews
- 2 teaspoons of lemon juice
- 3 tablespoon of olive oil, divided
- 8-ounce of tomato paste
- 4 fluid ounce of water

Directions:

1. Place the cashews in a food processor; add the garlic powder, 1/2 teaspoon of salt, yeast, 2 tablespoons of oil, lemon juice, and water.
2. Mash it until it gets smooth and creamy, but add some water if need be.
3. Grease a 4 to 6 quarts slow cooker with a non-stick cooking spray and insert the pizza crust into it.
4. Press the dough in bottom and spread the tomato paste on top of it.

5. Sprinkle it with garlic powder, oregano and top it with the prepared cashew mixture.

6. Spray it with the mushrooms, bell peppers, tomato, artichoke slices, olives and then with the remaining olive oil.

7. Sprinkle it with the oregano, the remaining salt and cover it with the lid.

8. Plug in the slow cooker and let it cook for 1 to 1 1/2 hours at the low heat setting or until the crust turns golden brown.

9. When done, transfer the pizza to the cutting board, let it rest for 10 minutes and slice to serve.

Nutrition:

Calories: 212 Cal,

Carbohydrates: 39g,

Protein: 16g,

Fats: 5g, Fiber: 5g.

Black Bean Pizza Plate

Preparation Time: 10 minutes

Cooking Time: 20 minutes

Serving: 2

Ingredients

- 2 prebaked pizza crusts
- ½ cup Spicy Black Bean Dip
- 1 tomato, thinly sliced
- 1 carrot, grated
- 1 red onion
- 1 avocado

Direction

1. Preheat the oven to 400°F.
2. Lay the two crusts out on a large baking sheet. Spread half the Spicy Black Bean Dip on each pizza crust.
3. Then layer on the tomato slices with a pinch pepper if you like. Sprinkle the grated carrot with the sea salt and lightly massage it in with your hands.
4. Spread the carrot on top of the tomato, then add the onion.

5. Pop the pizzas in the oven for 10 to 20 minutes, or until they're done to your taste. Top the cooked pizzas with sliced avocado and another sprinkle of pepper.

Nutrition

379 Calories

15g Fiber

13g Protein

Tangy Barbecue Tofu Pizza

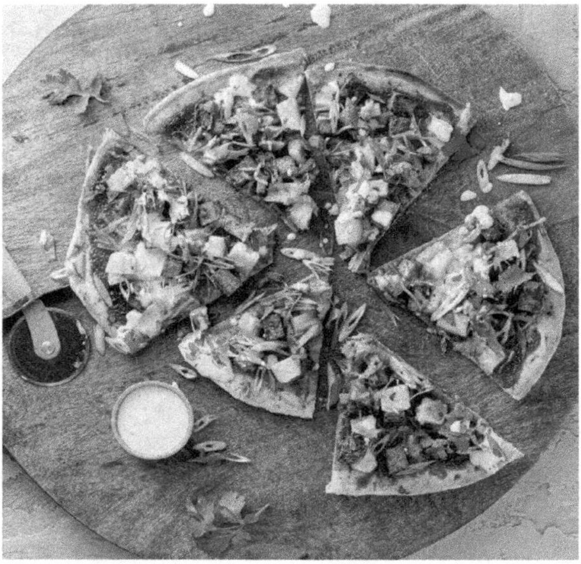

Preparation time: 20 minutes

Cooking time: 2 hours

Servings: 6

Ingredients:

- 12 inch of frozen whole-wheat pizza crust, thawed
- 1 cup of tofu pieces
- 1 small red onion, peeled and sliced
- 1/4 cup of chopped cilantro
- 1 1/2 teaspoons of salt

- 3/4 teaspoon of ground black pepper
- 1 tablespoon of olive oil
- 1 cup of barbecue sauce
- 2 cups of vegan mozzarella

Directions:

1. Place a large non-stick skillet pan over an average heat, add 1 tablespoon of oil and let it heat.
2. Add the tofu pieces in a single layer sprinkle it with 1 teaspoon of salt, black pepper and cook for 5 to 7 minutes or until it gets crispy with a golden brown on all sides.
3. Transfer the tofu pieces into a bowl, add 1/2 cup of the barbecue sauce and toss it properly to coat.
4. Grease a 4 to 6 quarts slow cooker with a non-stick cooking spray and insert the pizza crust in it.
5. Press the dough into the bottom and spread the remaining 1/2 cup of the barbecue sauce.
6. Evenly garnish it with tofu pieces and onion slices.
7. Sprinkle it with the mozzarella cheese and cover it with the lid.

8. Plug in the slow cooker and let it cook for 1 to 1 1/2 hours at the low heat setting or until the crust turns golden brown.

9. When done, transfer the pizza into the cutting board, let it rest for 10 minutes and slice to serve.

Nutrition:

Calories: 135 Cal,

Carbohydrates: 15g,

Protein: 6g,

Fats: 5g,

Fiber: 1g.

Tasty Tomato Garlic Mozzarella Pizza

Preparation time: 20 minutes
Cooking time: 2 hours 30 minutes
Servings: 6
Ingredients:

- 12 inch of frozen whole-wheat pizza crust, thawed
- 3/4 teaspoon of tapioca flour
- 2 teaspoons of minced garlic
- 2 teaspoons of agar powder
- 1 teaspoon of cornstarch
- 1 teaspoon of salt, divided
- 1/2 teaspoon of red pepper flakes
- 1/2 teaspoon of dried basil
- 1/2 teaspoon of dried parsley
- 2 tablespoons of olive oil
- 1/4 teaspoon of lemon juice
- 3/4 teaspoon of apple cider vinegar
- 8 fluid ounce of coconut milk, unsweetened

Directions:

1. Start by preparing the mozzarella.
2. Place a small saucepan over a medium-low heat, pour in the milk and let it steam until it gets warm thoroughly.
3. With a whisker, pour in the agar powder and stir properly until it dissolves completely.
4. Switch the temperature to a low and pour in the salt, lemon juice, vinegar, and whisk them properly.
5. Mix the tapioca flour and cornstarch with 2 tablespoons of water before adding it to the milk mixture.
6. Whisk properly and transfer this mixture to a greased bowl.
7. Place the bowl in a refrigerator for 1 hour or until it is set.
8. Then grease a- 4 to 6 quarts of the slow cooker with a non-stick cooking spray and insert pizza crust into it.
9. Press the dough into the bottom and brush the top with olive oil.

10. Spread the garlic and then cover it with the tomato slices.
11. Sprinkle it with salt, red pepper flakes, basil, and the oregano.
12. Cut the mozzarella cheese into coins and place them across the top of the pizza.
13. Cover it with the lid, plug in the slow cooker, let it cook for 1 to 1 1/2 hours at the low heat setting or until the crust turns golden brown and the cheese melts completely.
14. When done, transfer the pizza to the cutting board, then let it rest for 5 minutes, and slice to serve.

Nutrition:

Calories: 113 Cal,

Carbohydrates: 10g,

Protein: 7g,

Fats: 5g,

Fiber: 1g.

Burgers And Patties

Cauliflower Potato Burgers

Preparation time: 15 minutes

Cooking time: 7 minutes

Servings: 2

Ingredients:

- 7 oz cauliflower rice
- 1/4 cup mashed potato
- 1 tablespoon almond flour
- 1 teaspoon salt
- 1 teaspoon white pepper
- 1 tablespoon coconut yogurt
- 1 tablespoon breadcrumbs
- 1/2 cup water, for cooking

Directions:

1. In the mixing bowl combine cauliflower rice and mashed potato.

2. Add almond flour, salt, white pepper, and coconut yogurt.
3. Then wear gloves and make medium size burgers from the mixture.
4. Sprinkle every burger with breadcrumbs and wrap in the foil.
5. Pour water in the instant pot bowl and insert steamer rack.
6. Place wrapped burgers on the steamer rack and close the lid.
7. Cook the meal on High (Manual mode) for 7 minutes. Then allow natural pressure release for 10 minutes.

Nutrition:

Calories: 163,

Fat: 9,

Fibre: 4.8,

Carbs: 17,

Protein: 6.6

Sweet Potato Burgers

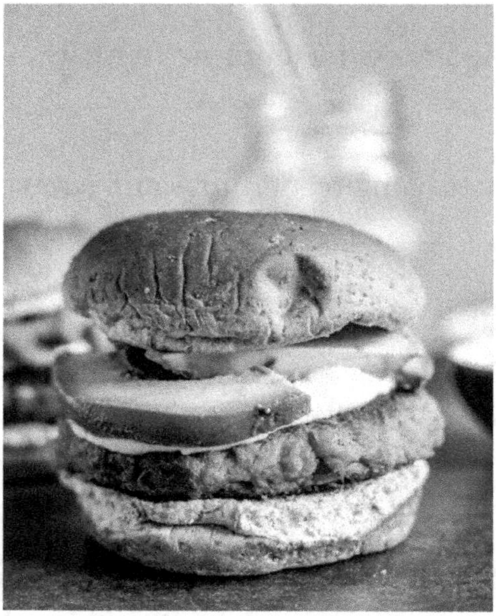

Preparation time: 10 minutes

Cooking time: 20 minutes

Servings: 2

Ingredients:

- 1 sweet potato
- 1/2 onion, diced
- 1 teaspoon chives
- 1/2 teaspoon salt
- 1 teaspoon cayenne pepper

- 3 tablespoon flax meal
- 1/2 cup kale
- 1 teaspoon olive oil
- 1/2 cup water, for cooking

Directions:

1. Pour water in the instant pot and insert steamer rack.
2. Place sweet potato on the steamer rack and close the lid.
3. Cook the vegetables on Manual mode (High pressure) for 15 minutes (quick pressure release).
4. Meanwhile, place onion, chives, and kale in the blender. Blend until smooth.
5. Transfer the blended mixture in the mixing bowl.
6. When the sweet potato is cooked – cut it into halves and scoop all the flesh into the kale mixture. Mix it up carefully with the help of the fork.
7. Add flax meal, salt, and cayenne pepper. Stir well.
8. With the help of the fingertips make medium burgers.

9. Clean the instant pot bowl and put olive oil inside.
10. Preheat for 2-3 minutes on Sauté mode.
11. Then add burgers and cook them for 2 minutes from each side on Sauté mode.

Nutrition:

Calories: 139,

Fat: 6.4,

Fiber: 6,

Carbs: 19.7,

Protein: 4.3

Potato Patties

Preparation time: 10 minutes

Cooking time: 15 minutes

Servings: 4

Ingredients:

- 3 russet potatoes, peeled
- 3 tablespoon aquafaba
- 1/2 teaspoon salt
- 1 teaspoon almond butter
- 1/2 teaspoon smoked paprika
- 1/4 teaspoon chili flakes
- 2 tablespoon wheat flour

Directions:

1. With the help of the hand mixer, whisk aquafaba until you get soft peaks.
2. Then grate potatoes and combine them together with aquafaba in the mixing bowl.
3. Add salt, smoked paprika, chili flakes, and wheat flour. Mix it up carefully.

4. Preheat the instant pot on Sauté mode for 4 minutes. Add almond butter and melt it.
5. Then with the help of the spoon make medium patties; press them little with the help of hand palms and put in the hot almond butter.
6. Cook the patties for 3 minutes then flip into another side. Cook the patties for 4 minutes more.

Nutrition:

Calories: 150,

Fat: 2.5,

Fiber: 4.4,

Carbs: 29,

Protein: 4

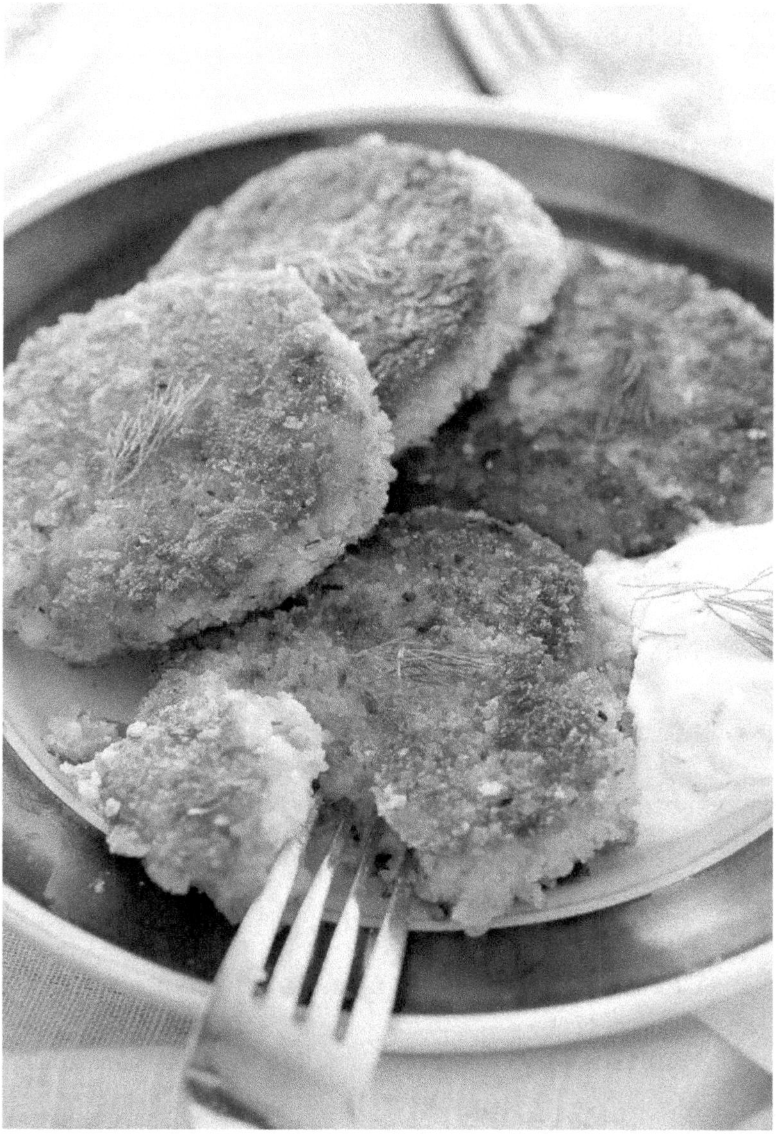

Lentil Burgers

Preparation time: 20 minutes

Cooking time: 26 minutes

Servings: 7

Ingredients:

- 1 cup lentils, soaked overnight
- 1 cup of water
- 1/2 carrot, peeled
- 1 teaspoon cayenne pepper
- 4 tablespoon wheat flour
- 1 teaspoon salt
- 1 teaspoon olive oil
- 1 tablespoon dried dill

Directions:

1. Put lentils to the Instant pot together with water, carrot, salt, and cayenne pepper.
2. Close the lid and set Manual mode (High pressure).
3. Cook the **Ingredients:** for 25 minutes and allow natural pressure release for 10 minutes.

4. Transfer the cooked **Ingredients:** in the blender and blend until smooth.
5. Add wheat flour and dried dill. Mix it up until smooth. If the mixture is liquid – add more flour.
6. Make the burgers and place them together with the olive oil in the instant pot.
7. Set Manual mode (High pressure) for 1 minutes (quick pressure release).
8. It is recommended to serve burgers warm.

Nutrition:

Calories 122,

Fat 1.1,

Fiber 8.7,

Carbs 20.7,

Protein 7.7

Black Beans Burger

Preparation time: 15 minutes

Cooking time: 5 minutes

Servings: 5

Ingredients:

- 1 cup black beans, cooked
- 2 tablespoons bread crumbs
- 1 teaspoon salt
- 1/4 cup sweet corn, cooked
- 1 teaspoon turmeric
- 1 tablespoon fresh parsley, chopped
- 1/2 yellow sweet pepper, chopped
- 1/2 cup of water

Directions:

1. Mash the black beans until you get puree and combine together with salt, sweet corn, turmeric, parsley, and sweet pepper.
2. Mix it up carefully with the help of a spoon.
3. Add breadcrumbs and stir again.

4. Pour water in the instant pot bowl and insert steamer rack.
5. Make the burgers from the black bean mixture and freeze them for 30 minutes.
6. Then wrap every burger in the foil and place on the steamer rack.
7. Close the lid and cook on Manual mode (High pressure) for 5 minutes.
8. Then allow natural pressure release for 5 minutes.
9. Remove the foil from the burgers and transfer on the plate. Garnish burgers with lettuce leaves if desired.

Nutrition:

Calories: 155,

Fat: 0.9,

Fiber: 6.5,

Carbs: 28.8,

Protein: 9.2

Mushroom Burger

Preparation time: 10 minutes

Cooking time: 14 minutes

Servings: 4

Ingredients:

- 2 cups mushrooms, chopped
- 1 onion, diced
- 1/2 cup silken tofu
- 1/2 teaspoon salt
- 1/2 teaspoon chili flakes
- 1 tablespoon dried parsley
- 1 teaspoon dried dill
- 3 tablespoon flax meal
- 1/2 teaspoon olive oil

Directions:

1. Put mushrooms in the blender and grind.
2. Then transfer the vegetables to the instant pot together with onion, and olive oil.
3. Stir gently and close the lid. Cook **Ingredients:** on Sauté mode for 10 minutes.

4. Meanwhile, mash silken tofu until you get a puree. Mix it up with salt, chili flakes, dried parsley, and dried dill. Add flax meal and pulse for 10 seconds.
5. When the mushroom mixture is cooked transfer it in the bowl and combines with the silken tofu.
6. Stir well.
7. Make the burgers.
8. Line the instant pot pan with baking paper and place burgers on it.
9. Close the lid and meal for 4 minutes on High. Then use quick pressure release.
10. Chill the burgers till the room temperature before serving.

Nutrition:

Calories: 47,

Fat: 2.6,

Fiber: 2.5,

Carbs: 5.4,

Protein: 2.6

Seitan Burgers

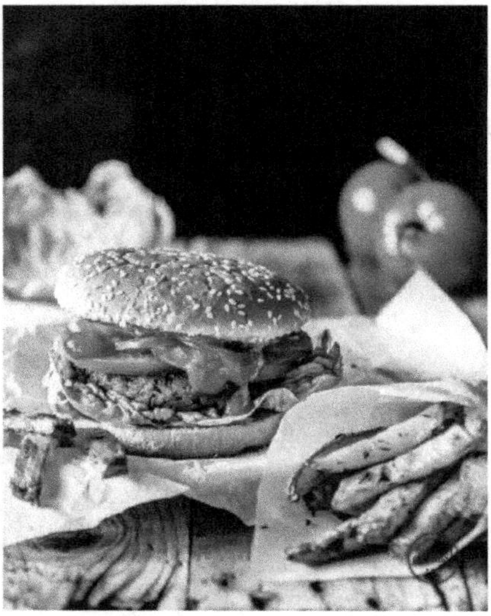

Preparation time: 10 minutes

Cooking time: 2 minutes

Servings: 1

Ingredients:

- 1 burger bun
- 1 teaspoon mustard
- 1 teaspoon soy sauce
- 1 seitan steak
- 1 teaspoon onion powder

- 1 teaspoon olive oil
- 1 tablespoon apple cider vinegar

Directions:

1. Make sauce for seitan steak: mix up together soy sauce, onion powder, olive oil, and apple cider vinegar.
2. Brush seitan steak with sauce from each side and place in the instant pot.
3. Close the lid and cook on Manual mode (High pressure) for 2 minutes (quick pressure release).
4. Meanwhile, cut burger bun into halves and spread with mustard.
5. Place seitan steak on the one half of burger bun and cover with the second one.

Nutrition:

Calories: 303,

Fat: 8.8,

Fiber: 2.8,

Carbs: 24.9,

Protein: 26.8

Spinach Burgers

Preparation time: 10 minutes

Cooking time: 10 minutes

Servings: 7

Ingredients:

- 3 cups spinach, chopped
- 2 tablespoon coconut shreds
- 4 tablespoon panko breadcrumbs
- 1 teaspoon salt
- 1/2 teaspoon chili flakes
- 2 tablespoon flax meal
- 6 tablespoon hot water
- 1 teaspoon olive oil
- 1 tablespoon coconut yogurt

Directions:

- In the mixing bowl mix up together flax meal and hot water. Whisk the mixture.
- Then add coconut shred, panko breadcrumbs, spinach, chili flakes, coconut yogurt, and salt.
- Mix up the mixture until homogenous.

- Set the Saute mode in Instant pot and preheat it until shows “Hot”.
- Then brush instant bowl with olive oil from inside.
- Make patties from the spinach mixture with the help of 2 spoons and place them in the instant pot.
- Saute them for 10 minutes. You can flip the patties during cooking if desired.

Nutrition:

Calories: 47,

Fat: 2.9,

Fiber: 1.3,

Carbs: 4.5,

Protein: 1.5

Tempeh Patties

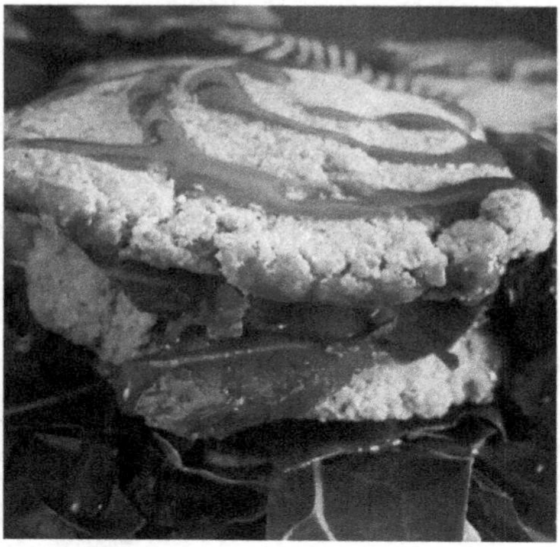

Preparation time: 15 minutes

Cooking time: 11 minutes

Servings: 5

Ingredients:

- 10 oz tempeh
- 1 carrot, peeled
- 4 tablespoon oatmeal
- 1/4 teaspoon minced garlic
- 1 teaspoon onion powder
- 1/2 teaspoon salt
- 2 oz black beans, canned

- 1 tablespoon tomato sauce
- 1 teaspoon golden syrup
- 1/2 cup water, for cooking

Directions:

1. Cut tempeh into the chunks and place on the steamer rack.
2. Pour water in the instant pot and insert steamer rack with tempeh.
3. Close the lid and cook on Manual mode (High pressure) for 7 minutes. Then use quick pressure release.
4. Meanwhile, chop carrot and place in the food processor.
5. Add minced garlic, oatmeal onion powder, salt, canned beans, tomato sauce, and golden syrup.
6. Blend the mixture for 2-3 minutes.
7. Then add cooked tempeh and keep blending for 1 minute more. The final mixture texture shouldn't be too smooth.
8. Use the burger mould and make burgers. Freeze them until solid.

9. Then wrap every burger in foil or use non-sticky paper and place in the cleaned instant pot bowl.
10. Cook the burgers on High (Manual mode) for 4 minutes. Then allow natural pressure release for 10 minutes.

Nutrition:

Calories: 175,

Fat: 6.6,

Fiber: 2.5,

Carbs: 18,

Protein: 13.7

Pumpkin Burgers

Preparation time: 10 minutes

Cooking time: 3 minutes

Servings: 2

Ingredients:

- 2 hamburger buns
- 1 tablespoon pumpkin seeds
- 1 tablespoon pumpkin powder
- 3 tablespoon pumpkin puree
- 2 tablespoons breadcrumbs
- 1/2 teaspoon chili flakes
- 1 teaspoon turmeric
- 1 tablespoon flax meal
- 3 tablespoons hot water

Directions:

1. In the mixing bowl combine flax meal and hot water. Whisk the mixture and add pumpkin powder, pumpkin puree, breadcrumbs, chili flakes, and turmeric.
2. Mix up the mixture. Add pumpkin seeds.

3. With the help of the burger mould, make 2 burgers.
4. Place them in the instant pot bowl and close the lid.
5. Set Manual mode (High pressure) and cook for 3 minutes.
6. Then use quick pressure release and open the lid.
7. Fill the burger buns with pumpkin burgers.

Nutrition:

Calories: 197,

Fat: 5.6,

Fiber: 3.3,

Carbs: 30.5,

Protein: 7.2

Bread Recipes

Strawberry Bread

Preparation Time: 15 Minutes

Cooking Time: 60 Minutes

Servings: 10

Ingredients:

- Eggs – 2
- All-purpose flour – 2 cups
- Vanilla – 1 teaspoon.
- Vegetable oil – 1/2 cup
- Baking soda – 1 teaspoon.
- Cinnamon – 1/2 teaspoon.
- Brown sugar – 1/2 cup
- White sugar – 1/2 cup
- Fresh strawberries – 2 1/4 cups, chopped
- Salt – 1/2 teaspoon.

Directions:

1. Preheat the oven to 350 F. Grease 9.5-inch loaf pan and set aside.
2. In a mixing bowl, mix together flour, baking soda, cinnamon, brown sugar, white sugar, and salt.

3. In a separate bowl, beat eggs, vanilla, and oil. Stir in strawberries.
4. Add flour mixture to the egg mixture and stir until well combined.
5. Pour batter into the prepared loaf pan and bake in preheated oven for 50-60 minutes.
6. Allow to cool for 10-15 minutes. Slice and serve.

Nutrition:

Calories 364,

Carbs 40.1g,

Fat 21.g,

Protein 4.2g

Moist Banana Bread

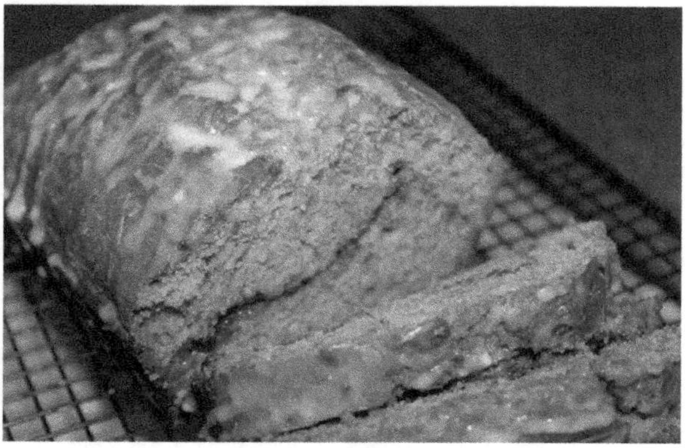

Preparation Time: 10 Minutes

Cooking Time: 60 Minutes

Servings: 6

Ingredients:

- Eggs – 2
- Baking powder – 1 teaspoon.
- Sugar – 1/2 cup
- Vanilla – 1 teaspoon.
- Vegan Butter – 1/2 cup, melted
- Ripe bananas – 3
- All-purpose flour – 1 1/2 cups
- Pinch of salt

Directions:

Preheat the oven to 350 F. In a large bowl, add bananas and mash until smooth. Add eggs, vanilla, butter, and mix well.

Add flour, baking powder, sugar, and salt and mix until well combined.

Pour batter into the greased loaf pan and bake in a preheated oven for 60 minutes. Slice and serve.

Nutrition:

Calories 388,

Carbs 54.6g,

Fat 17.3g,

Protein 5.9g

Banana Zucchini Bread

Preparation Time: 10 Minutes

Cooking Time: 45 Minutes

Servings: 12

Ingredients:

Eggs – 4

Cinnamon – 1 tablespoon.

Baking soda – 3/4 teaspoon.

Coconut flour – 1/2 cup

Coconut oil – 1 tablespoon.

Banana – 1, mashed

Stevia – 1 teaspoon.

Zucchini – 1 cup, shredded and squeezed out all liquid

Walnuts – 1/2 cup, chopped

Apple cider vinegar – 1 teaspoon.

Nutmeg – 1/2 teaspoon.

Salt – 1/2 teaspoon.

Directions:

Preheat the oven to 350 F. Grease loaf pan with oil and set aside. In a large bowl, whisk together egg, banana, oil, and stevia.

Add all dry Ingredients, vinegar, and zucchini and stir until smooth. Add walnuts and stir well. Pour batter into the loaf pan and bake for 45 minutes.

Slice and serve.

Nutrition:

Calories 78,

Carbs 4.4g,

Fat 5.8g,

Protein 3.4g

Broccoli Bread

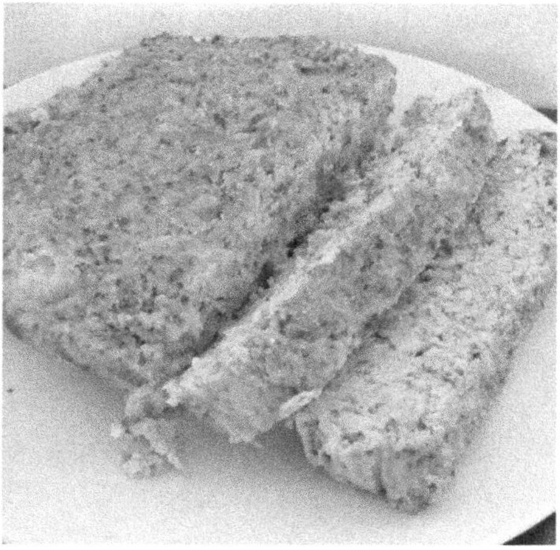

Preparation Time: 10 Minutes

Cooking Time: 30 Minutes

Servings: 5

Ingredients:

Eggs – 5, lightly beaten

Broccoli florets – 3/4 cup, chopped

Cheddar cheese – 1 cup, shredded

Baking powder – 2 teaspoons.

Coconut flour – 3 1/1 tablespoons.

Salt – 1 teaspoon.

Directions:

Preheat the oven to 350 F. Grease loaf pan with butter and set aside. Add all Ingredients into the bowl and mix well.

Pour egg mixture into the prepared loaf pan and bake for 30 minutes.

Slice and serve.

Nutrition:

Calories 205,

Carbs 8g,

Fat 13g,

Protein 13g

Almond Bread

Preparation Time: 10 Minutes

Cooking Time: 30 Minutes

Servings: 20

Ingredients:

Eggs – 6, separated

Cream of tartar – 1/4 teaspoon.

Baking powder – 3 teaspoon.

Vegan Butter – 4 tablespoons, melted

Almond flour – 1 1/2 cups

Salt – 1/4 teaspoon.

Directions:

Preheat the oven to 375 F. Grease 8*4-inch loaf pan with butter and set aside. Add egg whites and cream of tartar in a large bowl and beat until soft peaks form.

Add almond flour, baking powder, egg yolks, butter, and salt in a food processor and process until combined.

Add 1/3 of egg white mixture into the almond flour mixture and process until combined. Now add remaining egg white mixture and process gently to combine.

Pour batter into the prepared loaf pan and bake for 30 minutes. Slice and serve.

Nutrition:

Calories 52, Carbs 1g, Fat 4g, Protein 2g

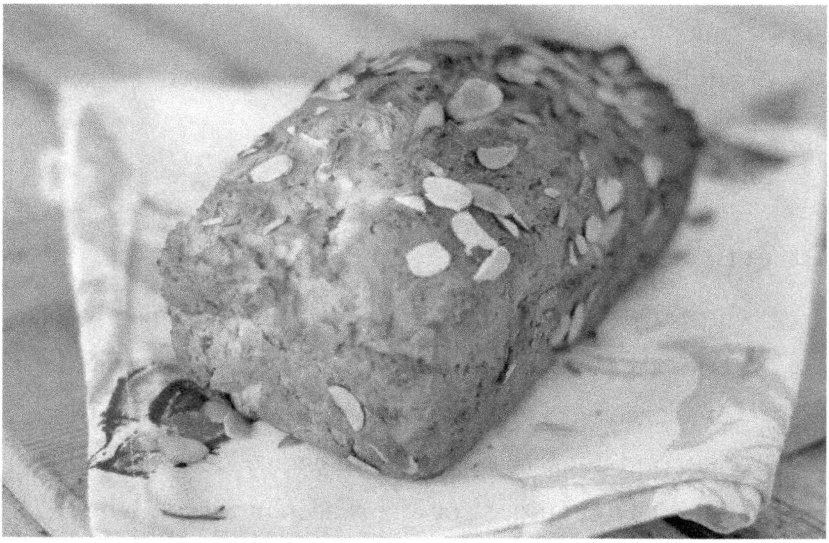

Sandwich Bread

Preparation Time: 20 Minutes

Cooking Time: 50 Minutes

Servings: 12

Ingredients:

Coconut flour – 1/2 cup

Apple cider vinegar – 1 teaspoon.

Water – 3/4 cup

Olive oil – 4 tablespoons.

Eggs – 5

Baking soda – 1 teaspoon

Almond flour – 2 cups + 2 tablespoons.

Salt – 1/2 teaspoon

Directions:

Preheat the oven to 350 F. Grease loaf pan and set aside. In a large bowl, combine together almond flour, baking soda, coconut flour, and salt. Set aside.

Beat eggs in another bowl until frothy. Add vinegar, water, and oil in egg mixture and process until well combined.

Add all dry **Ingredients:** and process until smooth. Pour batter into the prepared loaf pan and bake for 50 minutes. Slice and serve.

Nutrition:

Calories 125,

Carbs 2.5g,

Fat 11.5g,

Protein 4.7g

Sweet Rolls

Preparation Time: 2 hours

Cooking Time: 30 Minutes

Servings: 8

Ingredients:

2 tablespoons cane sugar

1 teaspoon rapid dry yeast

2 1/2 tablespoons warm water

1/2 cup pineapple juice, plus more for brushing tops of rolls

2 tablespoons coconut oil, melted

1 3/4 cups unbleached all-purpose flour, plus more for rolling out the dough

Directions:

In a small bowl, combine the sugar, yeast, and warm water. Stir gently and set aside for 10 minutes.

In another small bowl, combine 1/2 cup of pineapple juice and the coconut oil and stir.

Add the yeast mixture to the pineapple mixture and stir gently.

Add 1 3/4 cups of flour, and mix with your hands until well combined. The dough should not be too sticky. Knead in the bowl for 10 minutes, or until the dough is soft and smooth.

Place the dough in an oiled bowl, cover with a clean, damp towel, and place in a warm area for 1 hour to allow it to rise.

On a lightly floured surface, knead the dough, incorporating the flour from the surface. Break the dough into 8 equal pieces and form rolls.

Place the rolls on an oiled baking pan and allow to rise again for 30 to 40 minutes. Twenty minutes into this second rise, preheat the oven to 375 degree F.

Use a pastry brush to brush the tops of the rolls with pineapple juice.

Bake for 25 to 30 minutes or until golden brown.

Nutrition:

Calories 115,

Carbs 2.5g,

Fat 11.5g,

Protein 6.7g

Cornbread Waffles

Preparation Time: 6 Minutes

Cooking Time: 10 Minutes

Servings: 5

Ingredients:

1/3cup unsweetened plant-based milk

1 teaspoon apple cider vinegar

1/2 teaspoon baking powder

1/2 teaspoon baking soda

1 cup fine cornmeal

1/2 cup masa

1 cup unbleached all-purpose flour

1/3 cup unsweetened applesauce

1/4 cup sunflower oil

Coconut oil cooking spray

Directions:

In a small bowl, whisk together the milk and vinegar and set aside.

In another small bowl, whisk the baking powder, baking soda, cornmeal, masa, and flour together.

Add the applesauce and oil to the bowl containing the milk and stir to mix.

Pour the wet Ingredients into the dry Ingredients and whisk until well combined.

Turn a waffle iron on and coat with cooking spray.

When the iron is hot, pour in enough batter to fill the waffle iron and cook for 4 to 5 minutes, or until lightly golden brown.

Take the waffle out of the waffle iron and cut it in half. Repeat with the remaining batter

Nutrition:

Calories 175,

Carbs 2.5g,

Fat 9.5g,

Protein 5.7g

Buttermilk Biscuits

Preparation Time: 15 Minutes

Cooking Time: 15 Minutes

Servings: 8

Ingredients:

1 cup plant-based milk

1 tablespoon apple cider vinegar

2 cups unbleached all-purpose flour, plus more for cutting out the biscuits

1 tablespoon baking powder

1/2 teaspoon baking soda

1/2 teaspoon salt

1 tablespoon cane sugar

4 tablespoons (1/2 stick) Earth Balance vegan butter, cold

Directions:

Preheat the oven to 450 degree F and line a baking pan with parchment paper.

In a small bowl, mix the milk and vinegar and allow to curdle, usually no more than 5 minutes.

In a medium mixing bowl, whisk together the flour, baking powder, baking soda, salt, and sugar.

Add the cold butter and use your fingers or a pastry cutter to combine until only small pieces remain and the mixture looks grainy, like sand. Work fast so the butter doesn't get too soft.

Make a well in the dry Ingredients, and use a wooden spoon to stir gently while pouring in the milk mixture 1/4 cup at a time. Stir until well combined.

Sprinkle flour on a clean surface and dump the dough onto it. Dust the top of the dough with flour. Gently flatten the dough with your hands until it is about 1 inch thick, then dip a coffee mug rim into the flour to coat it and use it to cut out the biscuits.

Place the cut biscuits on the lined baking pan, and bake for 6 minutes, then turn and bake another 6 minutes or until the tops and edges turn golden brown.

Nutrition:

Calories 115,

Carbs 2.5g,

Fat 10.5g,

Protein 4.7g

Keto Cheese Bread

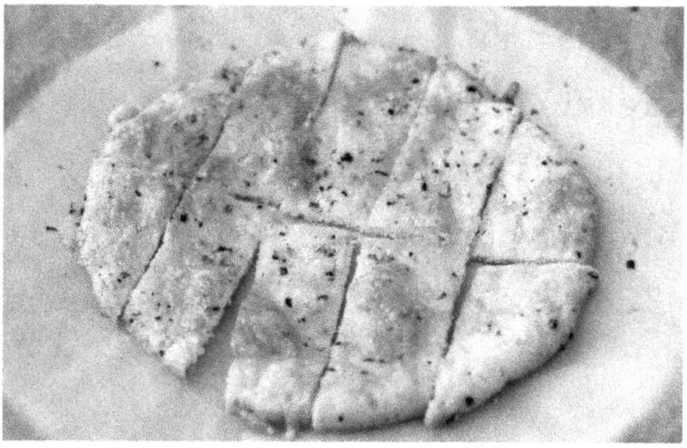

Preparation time: 9 minutes

Cooking time: 25 minutes

Servings: 6

Ingredients:

1 teaspoon Baking Powder

1/4 teaspoon Salt

1/3 cup Milk

1 cup Almond Flour

2 large Whole Eggs

1/3 cup Cream Cheese, softened

1/2 cup Grated Parmesan

Directions:

Preheat oven to 350 degree F.

Whisk together almond flour, baking powder, and salt in a bowl.

In a separate, bowl beat eggs and add cream cheese. Gradually stir in the milk.

Stir the wet mixture into the dry **Ingredients:**.

Fold in the grated parmesan.

Coat a 6-hole muffin tin with non-stick spray.

Divide the batter into the pan and bake for 25 minutes.

Nutrition:

Calories 203

Carbohydrates 6 g

Fats 16 g

Protein 9 g

Keto Mug Bread

Preparation time: 2 minutes

Cooking time: 2 minutes

Servings: 1

Ingredients:

1/3 cup Almond Flour

1/2 teaspoon Baking Powder

1/4 teaspoon Salt

1 Whole Egg

1 tablespoon Melted vegan Butter

Directions:

Mix all **Ingredients:** in a microwave-safe mug.

Microwave for 90 seconds.

Cool for 2 minutes.

Nutrition:

Calories 416

Carbohydrates 8 g

Fats 37 g

Protein 15 g

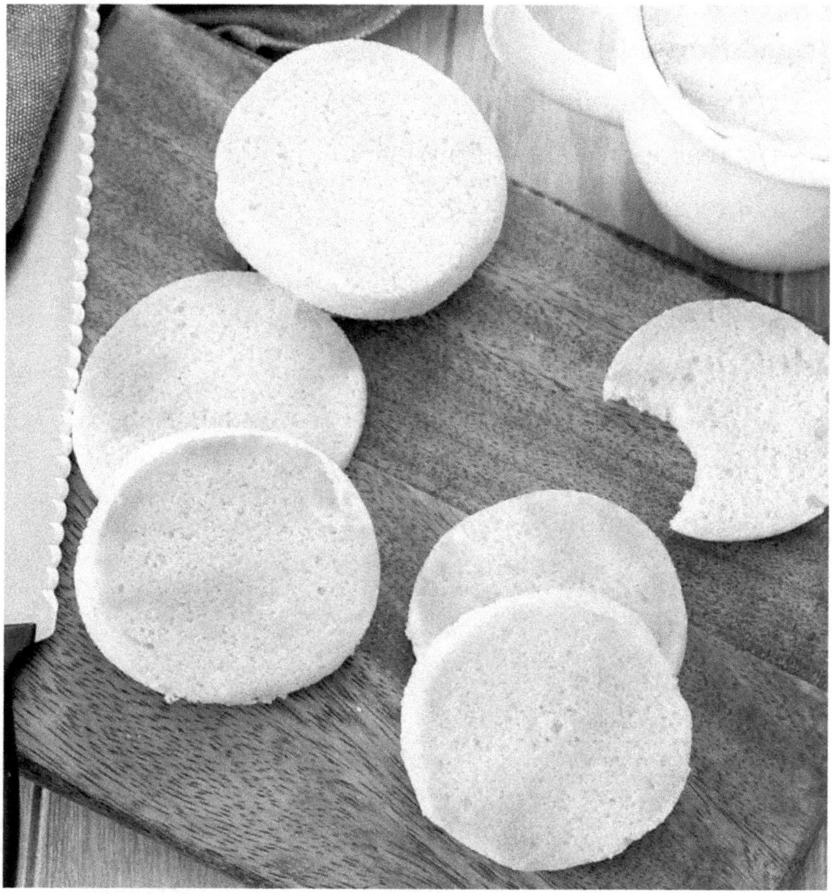

Keto Blender Buns

Preparation time: 5 minutes

Cooking time: 25 minutes

Servings: 6

Ingredients:

4 Whole Eggs

1/4 cup Melted Butter

1/2 teaspoon Salt

1/2 cup Almond Flour

1 teaspoon Italian Spice Mix

Directions:

Preheat oven to 425 degree F.

Pulse all **Ingredients:** in a blender.

Divide batter into a 6-hole muffin tin.

Bake for 25 minutes.

Nutrition:

Calories 200

Carbohydrates 2 g

Fats 18 g

Protein 8 g

Keto Burger Buns

Preparation time: 10 minutes

Cooking time: 12 minutes

Servings: 6

Ingredients:

1 cup Almond Flour

1/4 cup Psyllium Husk Powder

1 teaspoon Baking Powder

1 cup Mozzarella Cheese

1/4 cup Cream Cheese

1 Egg

tablespoon Sesame Seeds

Directions:

Preheat oven to 400 degree F.

Melt the two cheeses together in the microwave.

Blend the melted cheese together then stir in the egg.

Whisk together the almond flour, psyllium husk, and baking powder in a separate bowl.

Mix the dry **Ingredients:** into the cheese mixture until a dough is formed.

Divide the dough into 6 and roll each portion into a ball.

Top each ball with sesame seeds.

Arrange on a baking sheet lined with parchment and bake for 12 minutes.

Leave to cool for 10-15 minutes before slicing into halves.

Nutrition:

Calories 216

Carbohydrates 5 g

Fats 18 g

Protein 10 g

Keto Pizza Crust

Preparation time: 10 minutes

Cooking time: 6 minutes

Servings: 8

Ingredients:

1 cup Almond Flour

2 cups Shredded Mozzarella

2 tablespoon Cream Cheese

Pinch of Salt

Directions:

Combine both cheeses in a bowl and melt in the microwave.

Stir then gradually knead in the salt and almond flour.

Roll out to flatten in between sheets of parchment.

Bake at 350 degree F for 6 minutes.

Put choice of toppings on and bake for another 5-10 minutes.

Nutrition:

Calories 165

Carbohydrates 3 g

Fats 13 g

Protein 9 g

Coco-Cilantro Flatbread

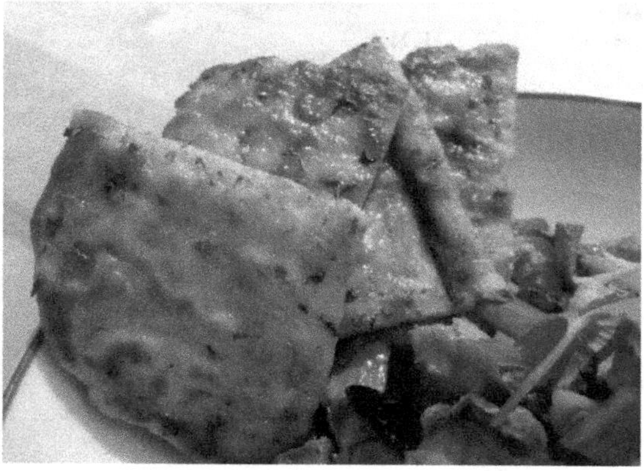

Preparation time: 10 minutes

Cooking time: 15 minutes

Servings: 6

Ingredients:

1/2 cup Coconut Flour

2 tablespoons Flax Meal

1/4 teaspoon Baking Soda

1 tablespoon Coconut Oil

2 tablespoons Chopped Cilantro

1/4 teaspoon salt

1 cup Lukewarm Water

Directions:

In a medium bowl, whisk together the coconut flour, flax, baking soda, and salt.

Add in the water, coconut oil, and chopped cilantro.

Knead until everything comes together into a smooth dough.

Leave to rest for about 15 minutes.

Divide the dough into 6 equal-sized portions.

Roll each portion into a ball, then flatten with a rolling pin in between sheets of parchment paper.

Refrigerate until ready to use.

To cook, heat in a non-stick pan for 2-3 minutes per side.

Nutrition:

Calories 46

Carbohydrates 1 g

Fats 4 g

Protein 1 g

Avocado Flatbread

Preparation time: 25 minutes

Cooking time: 5 minutes

Servings: 6

Ingredients:

130 grams Mashed Avocado

3/4 cup Chickpea Flour

1 teaspoon Cumin Powder

1/2 teaspoon Salt

Directions:

Combine all **Ingredients:** in a bowl. Stir until mixture comes together into a dough.

Knead the dough briefly on a lightly floured surface.

Leave the dough to rest for 15 minutes.

Divide the dough into four portions.

Take each portion of dough and flatten with a rolling pin.

Toast flatbread in a lightly oiled skillet for about 2 minutes per side.

Nutrition:

Calories 80

Carbohydrates 8 g

Fats 4 g

Protein 3 g

Keto Hamburger Buns

Preparation time: 5 minutes

Cooking time: 15 minutes

Servings: 5

Ingredients:

1 1/4 cup almond flour

1 1/2 cup mozzarella cheese, part skim grated

2 oz cream cheese

1 egg, large

2 tablespoons oat Fiber 500/ Protein powder

1 tablespoon baking powder

1 Metal plate or a pan which you care less about

Directions:

Using a microwave safe bowl, put the cream cheese and mozzarella cheese. Microwave the cheese for I minutes.

Remove the bowl, stir and microwave again for 40 seconds to another minute.

Scrape out the cheese and place it together with the egg into a food processor. Stop when it's smooth.

Add your dry **Ingredients,**processing it till dough is formed. (It is normally very sticky) Let the dough cool.

Preheat your oven to 400 degree F, placing the rack in the middle. Line your baking sheet with parchment paper and place the cheap metal plate or pan at the bottom of the oven.

Once the oven is ready, separate the dough into 5 equal portions. Apply oil on your hands (not too much) and roll the portions into balls.

Place them on the parchment paper, flattening them a bit while creating a domed shape.

Put 5 or 6 ice cubes on the metal pan and place the buns inside the oven. The steam from the cubes will make the buns rise.

Bake them for about fifteen minutes. They should be done once they brown on the outside. If not, give them more minutes in the oven.

Nutrition:

Calories 294

Carbohydrates 7 g

Fats 25 g

Protein 14 g

Paleo, Keto Buns

Preparation time: 10 minutes

Cooking time: 45 minutes

Servings: 10

Ingredients:

1 1/2 cup almond meal

1/2 cup coconut flour

1/2 cup flax meal

2/3 cup psyllium husks

6 egg whites, large

2 eggs, large

5 tablespoons sesame seeds

2 teaspoons garlic powder

2 teaspoons cream of tartar/ apple cider vinegar

2 teaspoon onion powder

1 teaspoon baking soda

1 teaspoon sea salt/ pink Himalayan

2 tablespoons Erythritol

480 ml boiling water

Directions:

Preheat your oven to 350 degree F

Mix all your dry **Ingredients:** in a mixing bowl.

Add your egg whites and eggs. Use a hand mixer to process it till your dough becomes thick.

Add the boiling water and process until it combines.

Line your baking sheet with parchment paper.

Use a spoon to make the buns and create a dome shape.

Sprinkle the sesame seeds on the buns. Press the seeds into the buns to prevent them from falling out.

Bake for 45 minutes.

Nutrition:

Calories 208

Carbohydrates 9 g

Fats 12 g

Protein 6 g

Low-Carb Coconut Hamburger Buns

Preparation time: 10 minutes

Cooking time: 20 minutes

Servings: 4

Ingredients:

1/2 cup coconut flour

1 1/2 cups mozzarella cheese, shredded

2 tablespoons cream cheese, softened

2 tablespoons flax meal

2 eggs, large

1 tablespoon baking powder

1 tablespoon sesame seeds

1/2 teaspoon salt

Directions:

Preheat your oven to 380 degree F.

Using a mixing bowl, whisk your flax meal, coconut flour, salt and baking soda.

In another bowl, put your cream cheese and mozzarella cheese. Microwave your cheese for 45 seconds to a minute. Stir it and microwave once more until it becomes melted.

Beat your eggs, adding into the first bowl which has the dry **Ingredients:**. Add the cheese too to the bowl. You can use your hand mixer to make the dough.

Separate the dough into four equal portions. Use these portions to make the buns and sprinkle sesame seeds. Press the seeds to prevent them from falling out.

Line the baking sheet with parchment paper and place your buns.

Bake for 20 minutes or until they brown on the outside.

Leave them to cool.

Nutrition:

Calories 218

Carbohydrates 7.2 g

Fats 13.5 g

Protein 17 g

Low-Carb Dinner Rolls

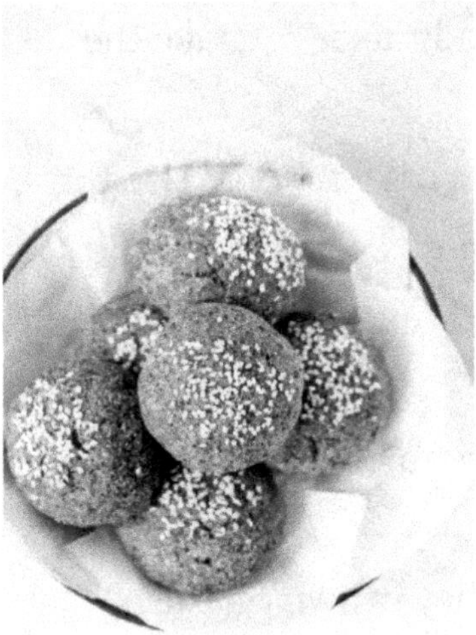

Preparation time: 10 minutes

Cooking time: 10 minutes

Servings: 6

Ingredients:

1 cup almond flour

1/4 cup flaxseed, ground

1 cup Mozzarella, shredded

1 oz cream cheese

1/2 teaspoon baking soda

1 egg

Directions:

Preheat your oven to 400 degree F.

Using a microwave-safe mixing bowl, microwave cream cheese and the mozzarella for a minute. Stir them till they become smooth.

Add eggs in the bowl while stirring to mix well.

In another clean bowl, put your almond flour, baking soda and flaxseed and mix the dry **Ingredients:**.

Pour your egg and cheese mix into the bowl with dry **Ingredients:**. Use your hand mixer or hands to make dough by kneading.

Slightly wet your hands with coconut oil or olive oil and roll your dough to six balls.

Top them with sesame seeds and place them on the parchment paper.

Bake them for 10 minutes. A golden brown look will indicate that they are done.

Leave them to cool.

Nutrition:

Calories 219

Carbohydrates 5.6 g

Fats 18 g

Protein 10.7 g

Keto Bread Rolls

Preparation time: 10 minutes

Cooking time: 20 minutes

Servings: 8

Ingredients:

1 1/3 cups almond flour

1 1/2 cups shredded mozzarella cheese, part skim

2 oz cream cheese, full Fat

1 1/2 tablespoon baking powder, aluminum free

2 tablespoons coconut flour

3 eggs

Directions:

Preheat your oven to 350 degree F

In a clean bowl, put almond flour, coconut flour and baking powder. Mix well and set it aside.

Using a microwave-safe bowl, put the cream cheese and mozzarella in it and microwave for 30 seconds.

Remove the bowl, stir and microwave again for 30 seconds. This should go on until the cheese has entirely melted.

Using a food processor add the cheese, the eggs and flour mix. Process at high speed for uniformity of the dough. (It is normally sticky.)

Knead the dough into a dough ball and separate it into 8 equal pieces. Slightly wet your hands with oil for this step.

Roll each piece with your palms to form a ball and place each ball on the baking sheet. (should be 2 inches apart)

In a bowl, add the remaining egg and whisk. Brush the egg wash on the rolls.

Bake for 20 minutes or until they are golden brown.

Nutrition:

Calories 216

Carbohydrates 6 g

Fats 16 g

Protein 11 g

Instant Pot

Oatmeal with Berries

Preparation Time: 25 minutes

Cooking Time: 0 minutes

Servings: 1

Ingredients:

- 1 2/3 cups water
- 1 cup quick oats
- 1 cup frozen berries
- 1 banana, chopped
- 1-2 tablespoon brown sugar
- 1/4 cup soy milk or almond milk
- 1-2 tablespoon brown sugar

For Garnishing (Optional):

- Almonds, chopped
- Coconut flakes

Directions:

1. Add water and oats directly to Instant Pot and cover it.

2. Switch on manual button for 6 minutes over high pressure. When the timer goes off allow the pressure to release naturally for about 10 minutes.
3. After 10 minutes, change the steam handle to 'venting'.
4. Open the lid and transfer the oats to a bowl and top it with mixed berries, banana, non-dairy milk and brown sugar.

Nutrition:

Calories: 200

Fat: 10

Fiber: 2

Carbs: 11

Protein: 15

Pumpkin and Oats Recipe

Preparation Time: 30 Minutes

Cooking Time: 0

Servings: 1

Ingredients:

- 1 cup steel cut oats
- 1 2/3 cups water
- 1 frozen banana
- 1/2 cup pumpkin purée
- 3 medjool dates, chopped
- 1 tablespoon of buckwheat groats
- 1 tablespoon of coconut flakes

Directions:

1. Add 1 cup steel cut oats to Instant Pot, along with water, pumpkin purée, banana, and chopped dates.
2. Stir it once and set steam release handle to 'sealing'. Switch on manual button for 10 minutes.
3. Once time is up, allow it for natural release for 10 minutes. Switch on 'Keep Warm/Cancel' button and change steam release handle to 'venting'.
4. Using a spoon, mix it around. Make sure to mash banana and dates together with oatmeal.
5. Serve it topped with some buckwheat groats and coconut flakes.

Nutrition:

Calories: 181

Fat: 15.2

Fiber: 4

Carbs: 10.8

Protein: 3.7

Strawberries and Cream Oatmeal

Preparation Time: 15 minutes

Cooking Time: 0 minutes

Servings: 4

Ingredients:

1 cup steel-cut oats

3 cups water

1 teaspoon strawberry extract

Vanilla-flavored nondairy milk

1 cup fresh strawberries, chopped

Directions:

Spray the instant pot with nonstick spray. Stir in the oats and water, then seal the lid and cook on high 3 minutes.

Let the pressure release naturally, then stir in the vanilla milk and fresh strawberries.

Nutrition:

Calories: 695

Fat: 66.7

Fiber: 11.1

Carbs: 22

Protein: 14.3

Pecan Pumpkin Spice Oatmeal

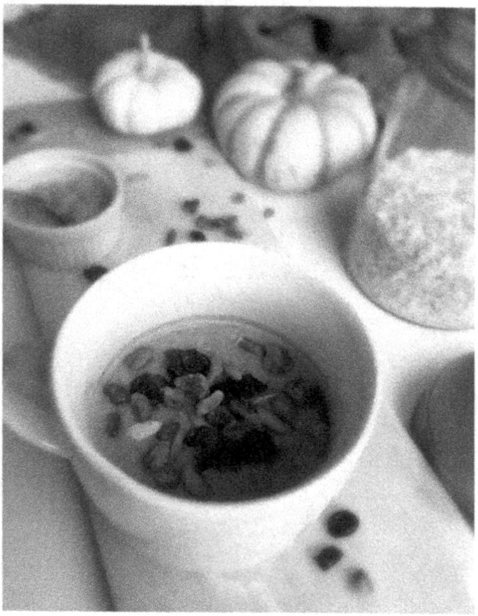

Preparation Time: 15 minutes

Cooking Time: 0 minutes

Servings: 2

Ingredients:

1/2 cup steel-cut oats

1/2 cup pumpkin purée

1 1/2 cups unsweetened almond milk

1/2 teaspoon cinnamon

1/8 teaspoon nutmeg

1 teaspoon vanilla extract

1/8 teaspoon of ground cloves

1/8 teaspoon ginger

1/4 cup brown sugar

Chopped pecans, for serving

Directions:

Spray the instant pot with nonstick spray. Combine everything except for the brown sugar and pecans.

Seal the lid and cook on high 3 minutes, then let the pressure release naturally.

Stir in the brown sugar and top with chopped pecans.

Nutrition:

Calories 251

Carbs 16

Fat 6

Fiber 8

Protein 7

Carrot Cake Oatmeal with Cream Cheese Frosting

Preparation Time: 20 minutes

Cooking Time: 0 minutes

Servings: 2

Ingredients:

1 small white sweet potato, peeled and steamed

1 small carrot, grated

1/4 small zucchini, grated

1/2 cup steel-cut oats

1 1/2 cups nondairy milk

1/2 teaspoon lemon juice

1/2 teaspoon apple cider vinegar

1/8 teaspoon of salt

1/8 teaspoon ground cloves

1/8 teaspoon nutmeg

1/2 teaspoon cinnamon

2 tablespoons brown sugar

2 tablespoons maple syrup

1 1/2 tablespoons coconut oil

1 tablespoon water

Directions:

To make the cream cheese frosting, puree half of the steamed sweet potato in a food processor.

Add the maple syrup, water, coconut oil, lemon juice, and apple cider vinegar and puree until smooth.

Add more sweet potato if the mixture is not thick enough.

Spray the instant pot with nonstick spray. Combine the rest of the **Ingredients,**then seal the lid and cook on high 3 minutes.

Let the pressure release naturally. Add additional milk to the oatmeal if needed, and top each serving with a dollop of the cream cheese frosting.

Nutrition:

Calories: 300

Fat: 15

Fiber: 5

Carbs: 8

Protein: 16

Chocolate Walnut Oatmeal

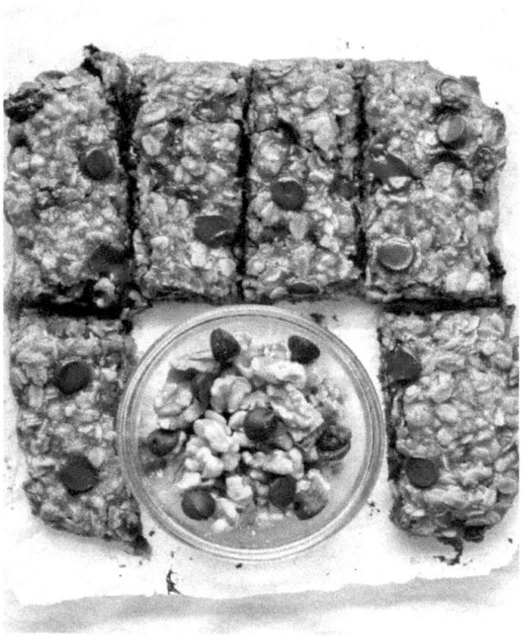

Preparation Time: 15 minutes

Cooking Time: 5 minutes

Servings: 2

Ingredients:

1/2 cup steel-cut oats

2 tablespoons cocoa powder

1 teaspoon brown sugar

1 tablespoon agave nectar

1 teaspoon vanilla extract

1/2 cup unsweetened almond milk

1 1/2 cups water

Semi-sweet chocolate chips, for topping

Walnuts for topping

Directions:

Spray the instant pot with nonstick spray. Combine the oats, cocoa powder, water, vanilla, brown sugar, and agave nectar.

Cook on high 3 minutes, then let the pressure release naturally. Stir in the almond milk.

Top with chocolate chips and walnuts.

Nutrition:

Calories: 275

Fat: 16.5

Fiber: 4.3

Carbs: 17.2

Protein: 17.4

Breakfast Burrito Filling

Preparation Time: 15 minutes

Cooking Time: 5 minutes

Servings: 4

Ingredients:

15 ounces tofu, drained and crumbled

1/2 cup water

1 clove garlic, minced

1/2 bell pepper, chopped

1/2 teaspoon chili powder

1/4 teaspoon chipotle chili powder

1/4 teaspoon sriracha sauce

1 teaspoon lime juice

Salt and pepper, to taste

1/4 cup shredded vegan cheddar cheese, for serving

Warm tortillas, for serving

Salsa, for serving

Directions:

Combine all the **Ingredients:** in the instant pot. Seal the lid and cook on high 4 minutes, then let the pressure release naturally.

If the mixture is too wet, drain off some of the water. Stir in the cheese to melt it. Serve wrapped warm tortillas with salsa.

Nutrition:

Calories: 186

Fat: 17.1

Fiber: 0.8

Carbs: 1.8

Protein: 7.4

Tofu Breakfast Custard and Potatoes

Preparation Time: 25 minutes

Cooking Time: 2 minutes

Servings: 4

Ingredients:

12 ounces frozen hash browns

1 shallot, chopped

2 tablespoons vegan chicken-flavored bouillon

10 ounces silken tofu

1/2 cup shredded vegan cheddar cheese

1/2 cup nondairy milk

1/4 teaspoon onion powder

1/8 teaspoon garlic powder

1/2 teaspoon seasoned salt

1/4 teaspoon freshly ground pepper

1 tablespoon olive oil

Hot sauce, for serving

Directions:

Puree the tofu, milk, bouillon, garlic powder, onion powder and seasoned salt in a food processor.

Heat the oil in the instant pot on the sauté setting and cook the shallot for 3 minutes.

Spread the hash browns on top of the cooked shallots, and top with the cheese.

Pour the tofu puree over the top, then sprinkle with fresh ground pepper.

Cook on high 5 minutes, then quick release the pressure.

The tofu mixture should be a jiggly custard texture. If it is too moist, return the instant pot to the sauté setting and cook longer with the lid on but vented.

Serve with hot sauce!

Nutrition:

Calories: 224

Fat: 19g

Protein: 18g,Carbohydrates: 0g

Apple and Sausage French Toast Casserole

Preparation Time: 25 minutes

Cooking Time: 5 minutes

Servings: 4

Ingredients:

4 links vegan breakfast sausages, chopped into coins

2 apples, peeled and chopped

Juice of 1/2 lemon

Zest of 1/2 lemon

1/2 loaf whole wheat bread, chopped into cubes

1 1/2 cups water

1 teaspoon vanilla extract

3 tablespoons unsweetened applesauce

1/2 teaspoon cinnamon

1 tablespoon olive oil

Maple syrup, for serving

Directions:

Heat olive oil in the instant pot using the sauté setting. Add the sausage and cook for 10 minutes.

Add the water, applesauce, vanilla extract, lemon juice, and cinnamon to the instant pot.

Add the apples, then the bread cubes. Push the bread down to make sure it is all coated with the mixture.

Seal the lid and cook on high 4 minutes, then let the pressure release naturally. Dust with powdered sugar and lemon zest and serve.

Nutrition:

Calories: 327

Fat: 25g

Protein: 36g

Carbohydrates: 0.3g

Granola.

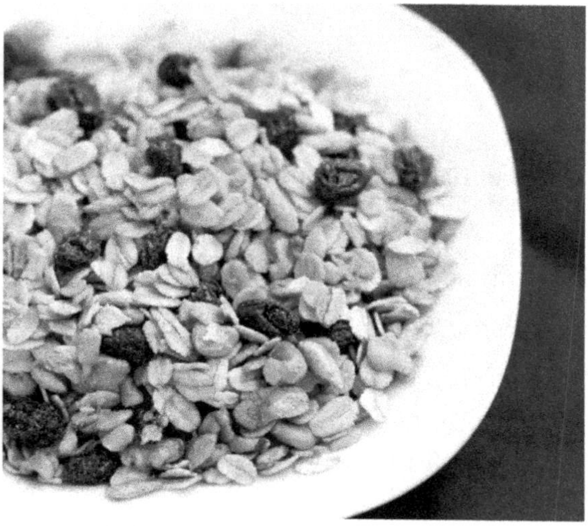

Preparation Time: 25 minutes

Cooking Time: 5 minutes

Servings: 8

Ingredients:

- 5 cups old-fashioned rolled oats
- 1 cup slivered blanched almonds
- 2/3 cup pure maple syrup
- 1/2 cup wheat germ
- 1/2 cup unsweetened shredded coconut
- 1/2 cup sunflower seeds
- 1/2 cup golden raisins or sweetened dried cranberries
- 1/2 cup chopped dates or dried apricots
- 1/4 cup vegetable oil

1/4 cup packed light brown sugar

3 tablespoons water

1 teaspoon pure vanilla extract

Directions:

Spray the Instant Pot insert with cooking spray and set to high.

Add the maple syrup, oil, water, sugar, and vanilla.

In a bowl combine the oats, wheat germ, almonds, sunflower seeds, coconut, and dates.

Mix the oats into the syrup mix in the Instant Pot.

Seal and cook for 12 minutes.

Release the pressure and cook with the lid open until your granola is crisp.

Nutrition:

Calories: 332

Fat: 12g

Protein: 34g

Carbohydrates: 0g

Spiced Apple Oats.

Preparation Time: 10 minutes

Cooking Time: 40 minutes

Servings: 4

Ingredients:

3 cups water

2 cups apple juice

2 apples, peeled, cored, and chopped

1 1/4 cups steel-cut oats

1/2 cup golden raisins or dried cranberries

1/4 cup packed light brown sugar or granulated natural sugar, or more to taste

1 tablespoon ground flaxseed

1 teaspoon ground cinnamon

1/2 teaspoon salt

Directions:

Lightly oil your Instant Pot insert with cooking spray.

Combine the Ingredients.

Seal and cook on Stew for 40 minutes.

Nutrition:

Calories: 200

Fat: 9g

Protein: 4g

Carbohydrates: 28g

PB&J Oats.

Preparation Time: 10 minutes

Cooking Time: 40 minutes

Servings: 6

Ingredients:

- 5 1/2 cups water
- 1 1/2 cups steel-cut oats
- 1/2 cup strawberry jam
- 1/2 cup creamy peanut butter, at room temperature
- 1 teaspoon ground cinnamon
- 3/4 teaspoon salt

Directions:

- Lightly oil your Instant Pot insert with cooking spray.
- Combine the oats, water, cinnamon, and salt.
- Seal and cook on Stew for 40 minutes.
- Release the pressure naturally and stir in the peanut butter and jam.

Nutrition:

Calories: 359

Fat: 18g

Protein: 15g

Carbohydrates: 21g

Conclusion

In a nutshell, this cookbook offers you a world full of options to diversify your plant-based menu. People on this diet are usually seen struggling to choose between healthy food and flavor but, soon, they run out of the options. The selection of 250 recipes in this book is enough to adorn your dinner table with flavorsome, plant-based meals every day. Give each recipe a good read and try them out in the kitchen. You will experience tempting aromas and binding flavors every day.

The book is conceptualized with the idea of offering you a comprehensive view of a plant-based diet and how it can benefit the body. You may find the shift sudden, especially if you are a die-hard fan of non-vegetarian items. But you need not give up anything that you love. Eat everything in moderation.

The next step is to start experimenting with the different recipes in this book and see which ones are your favorites. Everyone has their favorite food, and you will surely find several of yours in this book. Start with breakfast and work your way through. You will be pleasantly surprised at how tasty a vegan meal really can be.

You will love reading this book, as it helps you to understand how revolutionary a plant-based diet can be. It will help you to make informed decisions as you move toward greater change for the greater good. What are you waiting for? Have you begun your journey on the path of the plant-based diet yet? If you haven't, do it now!

Now you have everything you need to get started making budget-friendly, healthy plant-based recipes. Just follow your basic shopping list and follow your meal plan to get started! It's easy to switch over to a plant-based diet if you have your meals planned out and temptation locked away. Don't forget to clean out your kitchen before starting, and you're sure to meet all your diet and health goals.

You need to plan if you are thinking about dieting. First, you can start slowly by just eating one meal a day, which is vegetarian and gradually increasing your number of vegetarian meals. Whenever you are struggling, ask your friend or family member to support you and keep you motivated. One important thing is also to be regularly accountable for not following the diet.

If dieting seems very important to you and you need to do it right, then it is recommended that you visit a professional such as a nutritionist or dietitian to discuss your dieting plan and optimizing it for the better.

No matter how much you want to lose weight, it is not advised that you decrease your calorie intake to an unhealthy level. Losing weight does not mean that you stop eating. It is done by carefully planning meals.

A plant-based diet is very easy once you get into it. At first, you will start to face a lot of difficulties, but if you start slowly, then you can face all the barriers and achieve your goal.

Swap out one unhealthy food item each week that you know is not helping you and put in its place one of the plant-based ingredients that you like. Then have some fun creating the many different recipes in this book. Find out what recipes you like the most so you can make them often and most of all; have some fun exploring all your recipe options.

Wish you good luck with the plant-based diet!

CPSIA information can be obtained
at www.ICGtesting.com
Printed in the USA
BVHW091956220421
605650BV00002B/164

9 781801 834537